DIABETICS DIET AFTER 50

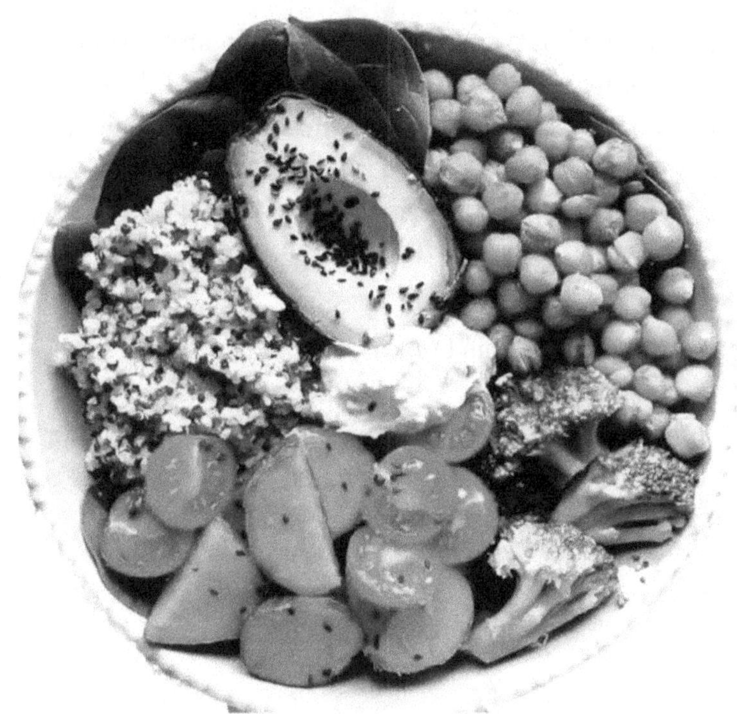

SUPER EASY DIABETIC DINING: EFFORTLESS AND DELICIOUS NUTRITION FOR VIBRANT LIVING AFTER 50

PATRICIA J. PETERSON

1

Contents

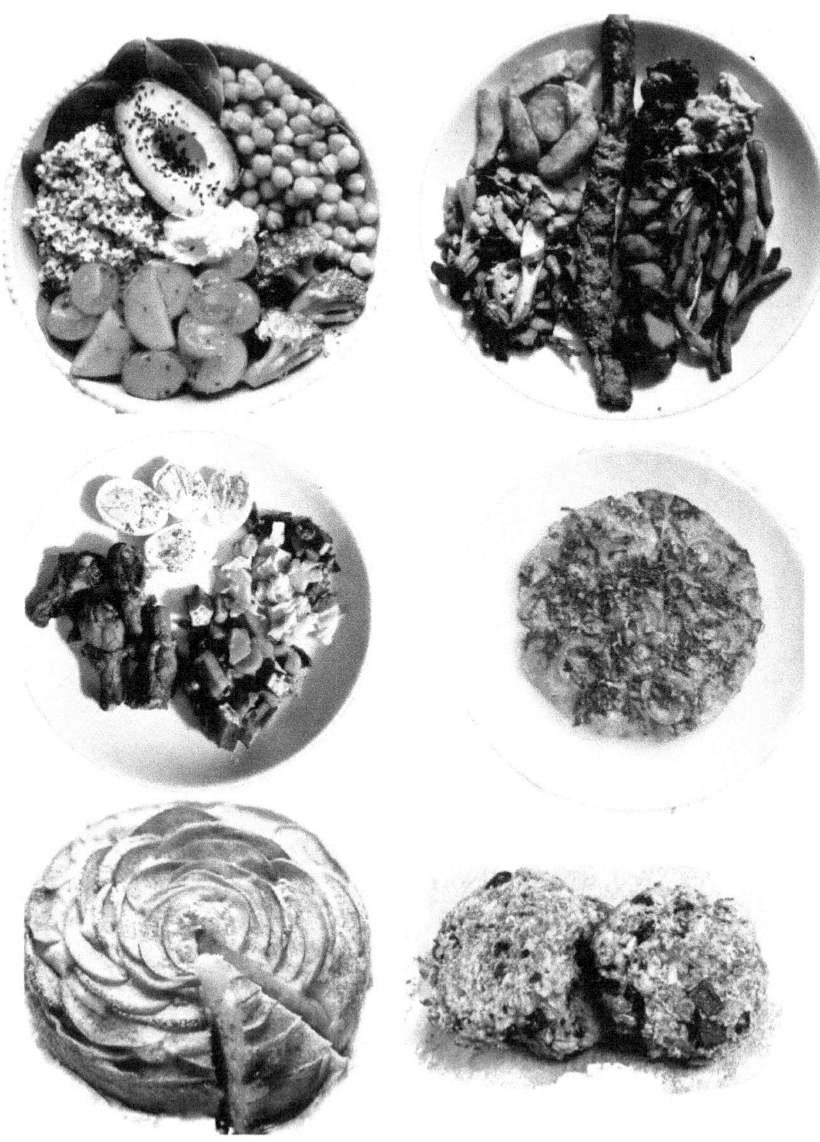

INTRODUCTION

Diabetes: Understanding Types, Causes, Symptoms, and Preventive Measures

Diabetes mellitus, or diabetes, is a chronic metabolic condition defined by increased blood glucose levels caused by abnormalities in insulin secretion, insulin action, or both. Insulin, a hormone generated by the pancreas, is essential in regulating blood sugar levels by enabling glucose uptake into cells. Diabetes develops when the body fails to produce enough insulin or grows resistant to its effects.

The chance of getting chronic health disorders increases as people age, and diabetes is one such major concern. Diabetes, which is characterized by increased blood glucose levels, necessitates close monitoring, particularly in people over the age of 50.

Diabetes Types:

Diabetes Type 1:

Type 1 diabetes is an autoimmune disease in which the immune system assaults and destroys insulin-producing beta cells in the pancreas.

Symptoms: Excessive thirst, frequent urination, unexplained weight loss, and weariness with rapid onset.

Because type 1 diabetes cannot be prevented, therapy entails lifetime insulin supply via injections or an insulin pump.

Diabetes Type II:

Type 2 diabetes: the most common type of diabetes in older persons, is frequently caused by insulin resistance and insufficient insulin production. Sedentary lifestyles, genetic factors, and obesity all play important roles.

Symptoms: Symptoms such as increased thirst, frequent urination, impaired eyesight, sluggish wound healing, and weariness appear gradually.

Preventive Measures: Lifestyle changes such as eating a nutritious diet, exercising regularly, and keeping a healthy weight can help to avoid or delay the onset of type 2 diabetes.

Gestational Diabetes

If a woman over the age of 50 becomes pregnant, she may still be at risk for gestational diabetes. Hormonal changes during pregnancy might cause insulin resistance, causing blood sugar levels to rise.

Symptoms: Although often asymptomatic, it is critical to monitor blood sugar levels throughout pregnancy.

Preventive Actions: Regular pregnancy check-ups, blood glucose monitoring, and living a healthy lifestyle can all assist control gestational diabetes.

Causes

1. **Changes with Age:** The aging process can have an impact on the efficiency of insulin generation and usage, raising the risk of diabetes.

2. **Genetics:** As we become older, our family history becomes increasingly important. Individuals who have diabetes in their parents or siblings should be cautious about their own health.

3. **Sedentary Lifestyle:** As we age, we lose physical activity, which adds to insulin resistance. Regular exercise has become critical for diabetes prevention.

4. **Obesity:** Changes in body composition are frequently associated with aging. Obesity,

particularly around the belly, is a significant risk factor for type 2 diabetes.

5. **Metabolic Syndrome:** As people age, they may develop a cluster of illnesses such as high blood pressure, high cholesterol, and abdominal obesity, which is known as metabolic syndrome and increases chance of developing diabetes.

6. **Medication Adverse Effects:** Certain drugs often provided for diseases such as high blood pressure may have an effect on blood sugar levels.

Common Diabetes Symptoms in People Over 50:

I. **Polyuria (Frequent Urination):** Changes in bladder function with age may exacerbate the symptom, necessitating close monitoring.

II. **Polydipsia (Excessive Thirst):** As we age, our bodies' ability to control fluid balance deteriorates, making excessive thirst more evident.

III. **Polyphagia (Excessive Hunger):** Changes in appetite and digestion might impact eating habits, necessitating strict dietary monitoring.

IV. **Weight Loss:** Unexplained weight loss in older persons may be an indication of diabetes and should be treated immediately.

V. **Blurred Vision:** Age-related eye changes may aggravate diabetes-related vision problems, stressing the importance of frequent eye exams.

VI. **Fatigue:** While aging causes fatigue, diabetes can exacerbate this condition, interfering with everyday tasks.

Diabetes Preventive Measures for People Over 50:

I. **Nutritional Balance:** A diet rich in whole grains, fruits, vegetables, and lean proteins is essential. To enhance general health, older folks should prioritize nutrient-dense diets.

II. **Regular Exercise:** It is critical to incorporate physical activity into everyday routines. Walking, swimming, and mild yoga can enhance insulin sensitivity and aid with weight management.

III.   **Weight Management:** Maintaining a healthy weight gets more difficult as we get older. It is recommended to consult with healthcare specialists for individualized weight management regimens.

IV.   **Routine health tests,** such as blood glucose, cholesterol, and blood pressure, are critical for early detection and management. Regular visits to healthcare providers should be prioritized for older persons.

V.   **Medication Administration:** People who use medications for diseases like hypertension or high cholesterol should be aware of the potential effects on blood sugar levels. It is critical to have regular contact with healthcare providers.

VI.   Diabetes can impair circulation and nerve function in the feet. To avoid issues, regular foot exams and adequate foot care are essential.

VII. **Stress Management:** Aging frequently brings with it new stressors. Adopting stress-reduction strategies, such as meditation or mindfulness, is beneficial to one's overall health and diabetes prevention.

VIII. **Social Support:** The emotional and social components of aging are critical to overall health. Participating in social activities and keeping strong support networks help to improve overall well-being.

Optimizing Health with a Diabetic Diet After 50: Foods to Include and Avoid

Individuals' health management becomes increasingly important as we age, particularly after the age of 50, especially for those with diabetes. A well-balanced diabetic diet is critical for maintaining good health, managing blood sugar levels, and avoiding diabetes complications. Here's a list of foods to include and avoid in a diabetic diet for people over the age of 50.

Food to be Include:

Grain Whole:

Include whole grains such as brown rice, quinoa, oats, and whole wheat bread in your diet. These grains have a reduced glycemic index, which aids in blood sugar regulation.

Vegetables and fruits:

Consume a wide range of colorful fruits and vegetables. They are high in fiber, vitamins, and antioxidants, all of which promote general health. However, because fruits contain natural sugars, moderation is essential.

Proteins that are low in fat:

Choose skinless fowl, fish, tofu, lentils, and beans as lean protein sources. Protein promotes fullness and helps to keep blood sugar levels stable.

Fats that are good for you:

Include avocados, almonds, seeds, and olive oil as sources of healthful fats. These fats promote heart health while also providing a consistent supply of energy.

Dairy or Dairy Substitutes:

Choose low-fat or fat-free dairy products or dairy alternatives that are calcium and vitamin D fortified. These are beneficial to bone health.

Foods High in Fiber:

Whole grains, legumes, fruits, and vegetables are abundant in fiber, which aids digestion, helps maintain a healthy weight, and stabilizes blood sugar levels.

Fish with a lot of fat:

Include omega-3-rich fatty fish such as salmon, mackerel, and sardines in your diet. These lipids are anti-inflammatory and beneficial to heart health.

Spices and herbs:

Use herbs and spices such as cinnamon, turmeric, and garlic, which may help manage blood sugar levels.

Foods to Avoid:

Carbohydrates that have been refined:

Reduce or avoid refined carbs such as white bread, sugary cereals, and pastries. These can result in fast blood sugar increases.

Sugary Drinks:

Avoid sugary liquids, such as soda and fruit juice. Instead, drink water, herbal tea, or sparkling water.

Foods that have been processed:

Reduce your intake of processed foods, which often contain hidden sugars, harmful fats, and high sodium levels. When possible, choose entire, unprocessed meals.

Snacks High in Sugar:

Limit your intake of high-sugar snacks such as sweets, cookies, and cakes. Instead, go for healthier snacks such as almonds or fresh fruit in moderation.

Fatty and fried foods:

Reduce your intake of fried and fatty foods, which can contribute to weight gain and have a bad impact on heart health. Select culinary methods such as grilling, baking, or steaming.

Excessive alcohol consumption:

Alcohol consumption should be limited since it can interfere with blood sugar management and may interact with diabetic treatments.

Trans and Saturated Fats:

Reduce your diet of saturated and trans fat-rich foods such as red meat, processed meats, and fried foods. Choose lean protein and healthier cooking oils.

Foods High in Salt:

Limit your sodium consumption by avoiding items that are very salty. High salt levels can contribute to hypertension, a prevalent problem in those over the age of 50.

Core Benefits of Following DIABETIC DIET

Controlling Blood Sugar:

A diabetic diet is intended to control blood sugar levels. It emphasizes the consumption of complex carbs, fiber-rich meals, and lean proteins, which help minimize blood glucose spikes and crashes. This is especially important for diabetics over the age of 50, as stable blood sugar levels contribute to overall well-being and lower the risk of problems.

Weight Control:

Weight management becomes more difficult as we age due to changes in metabolism and body composition. A diabetic diet promotes portion management, good food choices, and nutrient balance. This helps to maintain a healthy weight, which is vital for preventing insulin resistance and effectively controlling diabetes.

Cardiovascular Health:

Individuals over the age of 50 are more prone to cardiovascular problems, and diabetes increases the risk of heart-related illnesses even further. A diabetic diet high in heart-healthy fats and lean proteins yet low in saturated and trans fats promotes cardiovascular health. It aids in cholesterol management and lowers the risk of heart disease.

Digestive Wellness:

A diabetic diet that emphasizes fiber-rich foods including whole grains, fruits, and vegetables enhances digestive health. Fiber promotes regular bowel movements, prevents constipation, and helps maintain a healthy gut microbiota. This is especially crucial for the elderly, who may experience age-related digestive difficulties.

Health of the Bones:

Aging is connected with a decrease in bone density, and people over 50 may be more vulnerable to illnesses such as osteoporosis. A diabetic diet includes calcium and vitamin D sources, which are needed for bone health. This reduces the incidence of fractures while also promoting overall mobility and well-being.

Inflammation is reduced:

Chronic inflammation has been related to a variety of health problems, including diabetes complications. Anti-inflammatory foods, such as fatty fish, nuts, and antioxidant-rich fruits, can help reduce inflammation in a diabetic diet. This is advantageous for reducing diabetes-related inflammation and improving overall health.

Increased Energy Levels:

A diabetic diet's balanced and nutrient-dense composition provides a consistent source of energy throughout the day. Maintaining stable energy levels is critical for those over 50 in order to sustain daily activities, promote a more active lifestyle, and improve overall quality of life.

Improved Blood Pressure Control:

Hypertension is a prevalent problem among the elderly and diabetics. A diabetic diet's low-sodium and heart-healthy components aid in blood pressure management. This is critical for preventing diabetes and high blood pressure issues.

Improved Cognitive Function:

According to certain studies, diabetes and cognitive deterioration are linked. A diabetic diet's nutrients, notably omega-3 fatty acids found in fatty fish and antioxidants found in fruits and vegetables, may lead to improved cognitive performance. This is critical for preserving mental clarity and lowering the risk of age-related cognitive decline.

Medication Management Assistance:

A well-planned diabetic diet can help regulate blood sugar levels in addition to diabetes treatments. Adherence to a diabetic diet on a regular basis may reduce the need for higher medication doses, lowering the risk of adverse effects and encouraging improved overall health.

CHAPTER TWO

HOW TO STICK TO A DIABETIC DIET

Recognize Carbohydrate Counting:

Learn to count carbohydrates because they have a direct impact on blood sugar levels. Concentrate on complex carbohydrates like whole grains, legumes, and veggies. Distribute carbohydrates equally throughout the day to keep blood sugar levels stable.

Portion control should be prioritized:

To avoid overeating, keep portion proportions in mind. Use smaller dishes, portion control, and prevent second helpings. Portion control is essential for weight management, which is a critical aspect in diabetes management after the age of 50.

Select High-Fiber Foods:

Include fiber-rich foods like whole grains, fruits, vegetables, and legumes in your diet. Fiber aids in the regulation of blood sugar levels, the health of the digestive tract, and the sensation of fullness.

Incorporate Lean Proteins:

To preserve muscle mass and improve general health, choose lean protein sources. Choose skinless poultry, fish, tofu, lentils, and low-fat dairy products. Protein also helps to keep blood sugar levels stable.

Choose Healthy Fats:

Healthy fats, such as those found in avocados, nuts, seeds, and olive oil, should be prioritized. These fats are good for your heart and give a consistent supply of energy. Limit your consumption of saturated and trans fats found in processed and fried meals.

Limit your intake of refined sugars and processed foods:

Reduce your intake of refined sugars and processed carbs. These can result in fast blood sugar increases. For higher nutritional content, choose whole, unprocessed foods.

Limit Your Sodium Consumption:

Control your sodium consumption to improve your heart health. Instead of using too much salt to flavor recipes, use fresh herbs and spices. Be wary of processed foods, which can have excessive salt levels.

Keep Hydrated:

Stay hydrated throughout the day. Adequate hydration is critical for general health and can aid with blood sugar management. Limit your intake of sugary beverages and instead drink water, herbal tea, or sparkling water.

Plan Healthy Meals:

Make well-balanced meals using a range of dietary categories. Each meal should contain a combination of carbohydrates, proteins, and fats. This equilibrium promotes healthy energy levels and general nutrition.

Regular Meal Schedule:

To control blood sugar levels, stick to a steady eating routine. Divide your meals and snacks evenly throughout the day. To avoid blood sugar changes, avoid fasting for extended periods of time.

Keep an eye on your blood sugar levels:

Monitor your blood sugar levels on a regular basis, as directed by your healthcare provider. This allows you to measure the effect of various foods on your blood sugar and make dietary changes as needed.

Include Physical Activity:

Regular physical exercise supplements the effects of a diabetic diet. Exercise improves insulin sensitivity, weight management, and overall well-being. Before beginning a new workout plan, consult with your healthcare physician.

Prepare Yourself:

Keep up to date on nutrition, diabetes control, and lifestyle variables. Attend instructional seminars, read credible sources, and join support groups to improve your knowledge and confidence in treating diabetes after the age of 50.

Adapt to Changing Requirements:

Recognize that your nutritional requirements may change throughout time. Reassess your diet with healthcare providers on a regular basis to account for changes in health, medications, or lifestyle.

20 Healthy Ingredients to Include in your Shopping List.

1. **Grain Whole:**
   Whole grains such as quinoa, brown rice, oats, and whole wheat bread are ideal. These give fiber, vitamins, and minerals without producing blood sugar surges.
2. **Greens with a lot of leaves:**
   Include nutrient-dense leafy greens like spinach, kale, and collard greens in your diet. These are strong in fiber and low in carbs, promoting general health.

3. **Vegetables in a Variety of Colors:**
Choose colorful veggies such as bell peppers, broccoli, carrots, and cauliflower. These give important nutrients while also adding taste to your meals.

4. **Proteins that are low in fat:**
Choose skinless fowl, fish, tofu, and lentils as lean protein sources. These options provide vital amino acids without a lot of saturated fat.

5. **Fish with a lot of fat:**
Include fatty fish such as salmon, mackerel, and sardines. These are high in omega-3 fatty acids, which promote heart health and lower inflammation.

6. **Seeds and nuts:**
Almonds, walnuts, chia seeds, and flaxseeds are all good additions. These contain beneficial lipids, fiber, and nutrients. Because of its high calorie density, portion sizes should be considered.

7. **Avocado:**
Avocados are a good source of monounsaturated fats, which are good for your heart. They are also high in fiber and vitamins.

8. **Berries:**
Berries such as blueberries, strawberries, and raspberries are ideal. These fruits have less sugar than others and are high in antioxidants.

9. **Yogurt from Greece:**

Choose plain, unsweetened Greek yogurt instead. It's high in protein and probiotics while being lower in added sugars than flavored varieties.

10. Eggs:

Eggs are a versatile and high-protein option. They are a good source of critical nutrients and can be prepared in a variety of ways.

11. Extra Virgin Olive Oil:

Extra virgin olive oil is ideal for cooking and salad dressings. It contains monounsaturated fats, which are good for your heart.

12. Onions and garlic:

These aromatic vegetables add flavor to recipes without adding a lot of calories. They may also have health benefits, such as anti-inflammatory qualities.

13. Cinnamon:

Consider including cinnamon to your spice cabinet. It has the potential to reduce blood sugar levels and can be used to flavor both sweet and savory recipes.

14. Tomatoes:

Fresh or canned tomatoes with no added sugars are both versatile components. They can be included into salads, sauces, and soups.

15. Broth with Low Sodium:

For soups and stews, use low-sodium chicken or veggie broth. It enhances flavor without adding too much salt, promoting heart health.

16. Spices and herbs:

Stock up on herbs and spices like basil, thyme, turmeric, and ginger. They add taste without adding too much salt or sugar.

17. Flaxseed Dinner:

Flaxseed meal is high in fiber and omega-3 fatty acids. For an extra nutritional boost, add it to smoothies, yogurt, or baked goods.

18. Almond milk without sugar:

Unsweetened almond milk is a low-carbohydrate substitute for ordinary milk. It can be used in cereals, smoothies, and dishes.

19. Tea, Green:

Green tea is a low-calorie, hydrating beverage. It is high in antioxidants and may have health advantages.

20. Fruits with a Low Glycemic Index:

Fruits having a lower glycemic index, such as apples, pears, and berries, should be included. These fruits have a more gradual effect on blood sugar levels.

Complications of Diabetes in Seniors After 50 without a Proper Diet

Uneven Blood Sugar Levels:

Inadequate dietary management can cause fluctuating blood sugar levels, increasing the risk of hyperglycemia (high blood sugar) or hypoglycemia (low blood sugar). Seniors with diabetes are particularly vulnerable to these changes, which can lead to a variety of issues.

Cardiovascular Difficulties:

Diabetes already increases the risk of cardiovascular disease in seniors. Poor dietary choices, especially those high in saturated fats and processed carbohydrates, can amplify this risk, raising the incidence of heart attacks, strokes, and other cardiovascular issues.

Nerve Damage and Neuropathy:

Diabetic neuropathy is a common consequence, and seniors may have worse symptoms if their blood sugar levels are not well controlled. Numbness, tingling, and discomfort in the extremities can impair movement and quality of life significantly.

Nephropathy (Renal Impairment):

Diabetes makes aging kidneys more prone to its effects. Diabetes-related nephropathy can proceed without correct dietary controls, resulting in reduced kidney function and an increased risk of renal disease.

Retinopathy (vision complications):

Seniors are already vulnerable to age-related eye difficulties, and diabetes can exacerbate these challenges. Diabetes retinopathy is caused by poorly regulated blood sugar levels, which can lead to vision impairment and blindness.

Immune Function Impairment:

Diabetes patients who are becoming older may have a reduced immune system. Inadequate food choices can worsen this sensitivity, increasing the chance of infection and causing wound healing to be delayed.

Digestive System Issues:

Diabetes can cause digestive problems in seniors, such as gastroparesis, a condition in which the stomach takes longer to empty. A diet deficient in fiber and nutrients can exacerbate these gastrointestinal issues.

Skin Health Problems:

Skin issues, such as poor wound healing and an increased susceptibility to infections, are frequent in diabetic elders. Poor dietary habits might lead to poor skin health and delayed injury recovery.

Disorders of the Bones and Joints:

Aging people are more prone to bone and joint problems, and diabetes can exacerbate these disorders. Seniors may be at a higher risk of osteoporosis and osteoarthritis if they do not receive sufficient dietary support.

Imbalances in Hormones:

Diabetes can affect hormonal homeostasis, especially in the elderly. Poor dietary choices, such as an overabundance of processed carbohydrates, may contribute to insulin resistance, complicating hormonal regulation even further.

Impact on Mental Health:

Diabetes-related complications, together with the normal aging process, may have an impact on elders' mental health. Inadequate blood sugar management, aggravated by an unhealthy diet, can contribute to depression and anxiety.

Complications in Aging Women:

Female diabetic seniors may face extra problems, such as an increased risk of gestational diabetes during pregnancy, which can lead to complications for both the mother and the baby.

CHAPTER THREE

The Transformative Impact of Thoughtful Meal Planning on Diabetes Management After 50

1. Blood Sugar Management:

Meal planning allows seniors to schedule their meals with a focus on blood sugar control. Seniors can prevent blood sugar spikes and decreases by carefully selecting the types and amounts of carbs, proteins, and fats they consume.

2. Portion Management:

Maintaining a healthy weight is difficult for seniors, and portion control is essential. Meal planning aids in identifying appropriate portion sizes, limiting overeating, and promoting weight management—all of which are important aspects of diabetes care.

3. Nutritional Balance:

Meal preparation ensures a well-rounded and balanced nutrient intake. Seniors can combine a range of dietary groups, such as whole grains, lean meats, fruits, vegetables, and healthy fats, to acquire the vitamins and minerals they need.

4. Consistent Meal Scheduling:

Establishing a regular meal routine is useful for diabetic seniors. Consistent meal time helps regulate blood sugar levels and can improve medication effectiveness, resulting in better diabetes management.

5. Complication Prevention:

Proper meal planning can help prevent or reduce the risk of diabetic problems. Seniors can minimize their risk of cardiovascular disease, nerve damage, and other diabetes-related consequences by limiting their diet of carbohydrates, saturated fats, and sodium.

6. Weight Control:

Because of changes in metabolism and physical activity, it can be difficult for seniors to maintain a healthy weight. Meal planning helps with weight loss by providing scheduled and healthy meals, as well as diabetes control and overall wellness.

7. Better Digestive Health:

Seniors may encounter digestive difficulties as a result of aging and diabetes. Fiber-rich meals support digestive health and aid in the prevention of issues such as gastroparesis and constipation.

8. Increased Energy Levels:

Balanced meals with the proper ratio of carbohydrates, proteins, and fats help to maintain energy levels. This is especially crucial for seniors who may experience exhaustion, as it ensures they have enough energy for daily activities.

9. Medication Management Assistance:

Meal planning supplements medicine regimes. Seniors can properly plan their meals and prescriptions, increasing the effectiveness of diabetes drugs and lowering the risk of hypoglycemia or hyperglycemia.

10. Emotional Well-being:

Consistent and well-planned meals help with emotional well-being. Seniors can enjoy a varied and savory diet, which reduces the probability of feeling deprived, which is commonly connected with restricted diets.

11. Social interaction:

Meal planning promotes social interaction. Seniors can arrange and share meals with family and friends, which fosters a sense of connection and reduces isolation, all of which are key aspects of mental and emotional wellness.

7 –DAYS MEAL PLAN SAMPLE

S/N	BREAKFAST	SNACK	LUNCH	SNACK	DINNER
1	Scrambled eggs with spinach and whole-grain toast	Greek yogurt with a handful of mixed berries.	Grilled chicken salad with mixed greens, cherry tomatoes, cucumber, and a vinaigrette dressing	Carrot and celery sticks with hummus.	Baked salmon with quinoa and steamed broccoli
2	Whole-grain English muffin with avocado and poached eggs.	Handful of mixed nuts.	Lentil soup with a side of mixed green salad	Sliced cucumber with guacamole.	Grilled shrimp with asparagus and quinoa.
3	Oatmeal with sliced strawberries and a sprinkle of chia seeds.	Sliced apple with almond butter.	Quinoa and black bean bowl with grilled vegetables	Low-fat cottage cheese with pineapple chunks	Stir-fry turkey with colorful vegetables and brown rice.
4	Smoothie with spinach, banana, Greek yogurt, and a touch of	Cherry tomatoes with mozzarella cheese	Chickpea and vegetable curry with brown rice on the side.	Fresh berries with a dab of low-fat whipped cream	Baked chicken breast with sweet potato and green beans

	cinnamon			
5	Whole-grain waffle with sugar-free syrup and a small serving of mixed berries	peanut butter-covered celery sticks.	Tuna salad lettuce wraps with cherry tomatoes and olives	Orange slices with a handful of walnuts	Grilled steak with quinoa and roasted Brussels sprouts
6	Scrambled tofu with sautéed mushrooms and whole-grain toast.	A tiny apple and low-fat string cheese	Spinach and feta-stuffed chicken breast with roasted veggies on the side.	Greek yogurt parfait with granola and cut strawberries	Baked cod with lemon, brown rice, and steamed asparagus.
7	Smoked salmon, cream cheese, and cucumber slices on a whole-grain bagel.	A handful of almonds topped with dried apricots.	Quinoa salad with mixed beans, cherry tomatoes, and balsamic vinaigrette	Hummus on sliced bell peppers	Stir-fried vegetables and shrimp with cauliflower rice.

CHAPTER FOUR
HEALTHY AND SATISFYING BREAKFAST RECIPES

Omelette with Spinach and Mushrooms

Cooking Time: 5minutes | **Serving: 1**

Ingredients:

- Two huge eggs
- 1/2 cup chopped fresh spinach
- 1/4 cup sliced mushrooms
- Season with salt and pepper to taste.

Preparation:

- In a mixing dish, whisk together the eggs.
- Add the spinach, mushrooms, salt, and pepper to taste.
- Cook for 3-5 minutes in a nonstick skillet over medium heat.

Nutritional Information

- Calories: 250
- Protein: 18g
- Carbohydrates: 5g
- Fat: 18g
- Fiber: 3g

Greek Yogurt Parfait:

Cooking Time: Not required | Serving: 1

Ingredients:

- 1 cup plain Greek yogurt
- 1/2 cup mixed berries (blueberries, strawberries)
- 2 tablespoons chopped nuts (almonds, walnuts)
- 1 tablespoon chia seeds

Preparation:

- In a glass, layer yogurt, berries, almonds, and chia seeds.
- Layers should be repeated.

Nutritional Information.

- Calories: 300
- Protein: 20g
- Carbohydrates: 30g
- Fat: 12g
- Fiber: 6g

Breakfast Bowl with Quinoa:

Cooking Time: 2minutes | Serving: 1

Ingredients

- 1/2 cup quinoa, cooked
- A quarter cup almond milk
- 1 tablespoon shredded unsweetened coconut
- 1 tbsp. sliced almonds
- A half teaspoon cinnamon

Preparation:

- To make the quinoa, combine it with the almond milk, coconut, almonds, and cinnamon.
- Warm for 1-2 minutes in the microwave.

Nutritional Information

- Calories: 300
- Protein: 10g
- Carbohydrates: 40g
- Fat: 10g
- Fiber: 6g

Toast with avocado and smoked salmon:

Cooking Time: 5minutes | Serving: 1

Ingredients:

- 1 whole-grain bread slice
- 2 ounces smoked salmon
- 1/2 avocado, mashed

42

- To taste, lemon juice
- Black pepper

Preparation

> - Toast the bread.
> - Top with mashed avocado and smoked salmon.
> - Drizzle with lemon juice and season with black pepper to taste.

Nutritional Information

- Calories: 300
- Protein: 15g
- Carbohydrates: 20g
- Fat: 15g
- Fiber: 5g

Chia Pudding Overnight:

Cooking Time: Not Required | Serving: 1

Ingredients:

- Three tbsp chia seeds
- 1 cup almond milk, unsweetened
- A half teaspoon of vanilla extract
- Half-cup fresh berries

Preparation

> ➢ Chia seeds, almond milk, and vanilla extract are combined in a bowl.
> ➢ Refrigerate for at least 24 hours.
> ➢ Before serving, sprinkle with fresh berries.

HIGH IN FIBER, OMEGA-3, FATTY ACIDS, AND ANTIOXIDANTS.

Nutritional Information:

- Calories: 250
- Protein: 8g
- Carbohydrates: 30g
- Fat: 10g
- Fiber: 12g

Bowl of Cottage Cheese with Pineapple:

Cooking Time: Not Required | Serving: 1 bowl

Ingredients:

- 1/2 cup cottage cheese (low-fat)
- 1/2 cup pineapple chunks, fresh
- 1 tablespoon mint, chopped

Preparation:

> Combine cottage cheese and pineapple in a mixing
  bowl.
> Garnish with chopped mint.

**PROTEIN AND VITAMIN C ARE IMPORTANT
NUTRIENTS.**

Nutritional Information

- Calories: 200
- Protein: 15g
- Carbohydrates:
  20g
- Fat: 8g
- Fiber: 2g

Whole-Wheat Pancakes:

Cooking Time: 10minutes | Serving: 2

Ingredients

- Half cup whole-grain flour
- A half-cup almond milk
- 1 egg
- A half teaspoon baking powder
- A quarter teaspoon vanilla extract

Preparation:

➢ Combine whole wheat flour, sugar, baking powder, baking soda, salt, buttermilk, egg, and melted butter or oil in a mixing bowl.
➢ Stir into dry ingredients. Preheat a griddle or nonstick skillet, pour 1/4 cup batter onto each pancake, add desired extras, cook until bubbles appear and edges firm.
➢ Flip and cook second side until golden brown.

FIBER AND PROTEIN ARE ABUNDANT IN THIS DISH.

Nutritional Information:

- Calories: 200 (per pancake)
- Protein: 7g
- Carbohydrates: 25g
- Fat: 8g
- Fiber: 3g

Frittata with Vegetables:

Cooking Time: 8minutes | Serving: 1

Ingredients

- 2 eggs are used in this recipe.
- 1/4 cup chopped bell peppers
- 1/4 cup halved cherry tomatoes

- 1/4 cup crumbled feta cheese
- Season with salt and pepper to taste.

Preparation

- ➤ Whisk the eggs and throw them into a skillet.
- ➤ Cook until the vegetables are tender.
- ➤ Sprinkle with feta, salt, and pepper.

HIGH IN PROTEIN AND LOW IN CARBOHYDRATES.

Nutritional Information:

- Calories: 250
- Protein: 15g
- Carbohydrates: 10g
- Fat: 15g
- Fiber: 3g

Smoothie with Peanut Butter and Bananas:

Cooking Time: Not Required | Serving: 1

Ingredients:

- One banana
- 1 tbsp organic peanut butter
- 1/2 cup Greek yogurt, plain
- A half-cup almond milk

Preparation

> ➢ Blend all of the ingredients until smooth.

Protein, good fats, and potassium are all important nutrients.

Nutritional Information:

- Calories: 300
- Protein: 12g
- Carbohydrates: 30g
- Fat: 15g
- Fiber: 5g

Smashed avocado and tomato on rye:

Cooking Time: 5minute | Serving: 1

Ingredients:

- 1 medium tomato,
- sliced 1/2 avocado, mashed
- 1 whole-grain rye bread slice
- Season with salt and pepper to taste.

Preparation

> ➢ To begin, toast the rye bread.
> ➢ On the toast, spread the mashed avocado.
> ➢ Serve with sliced tomatoes on top.

> Season with salt and pepper to taste.

Nutritional Information

- Calories: 250
- Protein: 8g
- Carbohydrates: 30g
- Fat: 12g
- Fiber: 6g

Waffles with Almond Flour

Cooking Time: 15minutes | Serving: 1

Ingredients:

- 1/2 cup almond flour
- 2 eggs
- 1 tablespoon almond milk
- 1/2 tsp baking powder
- a quarter teaspoon vanilla extract

Preparation

> Preheat your waffle maker per the manufacturer's directions.

> In a large mixing basin, combine the almond flour, baking powder, and salt.

> Beat the eggs in a separate basin. Combine the melted butter (or coconut oil), almond milk, and vanilla extract in a mixing bowl.

- ➤ If you prefer a sweeter taste, stir with your preferred sweetener.
- ➤ Stir the wet ingredients into the dry ingredients until thoroughly incorporated. The batter should be thick but not too thick to pour. To prevent sticking, lightly lubricate the waffle iron with oil or cooking spray.
- ➤ Spoon the batter onto the hot waffle iron and spread it evenly.
- ➤ Close the waffle iron and cook for 4-5 minutes, or until the waffles are golden brown, according to the manufacturer's specifications.

LOW IN CARBOHYDRATES AND HIGH IN PROTEIN

Nutritional Information

- Calories: 200 (per waffle)
- Protein: 10g
- Carbohydrates: 5g
- Fat: 15g
- Fiber: 3g

Berry Almond Smoothie Bowl

Cooking Time: Not Required | Serving: 1

Ingredients

- 1 dish serves 1 person
- 1 cup mixed berries (strawberries, blueberries, and raspberries)
- A half banana
- A quarter cup almond milk
- 1 tbsp. almond butter
- 1 teaspoon chia seeds

Preparation:

- Until blended, combine berries, banana, almond milk, and almond butter.
- Pour into a bowl and sprinkle with chia seeds.

Nutritional Information

- Calories: 250
- Protein: 8g
- Carbohydrates: 30g
- Fat: 12g
- Fiber: 10g

Breakfast Burrito with Eggs and Veggies:

Cooking Time: 8minutes | Serving: 1

Ingredients

- 1 whole-grain tortilla
- 2 scrambled eggs
- 1/4 cup washed and drained black beans

- 2 teaspoons salsa
- 1/4 sliced avocado

Preparation

- ➢ Fill the tortilla with scrambled eggs, black beans, salsa, and avocado.
- ➢ Make a burrito out of it.

Nutritional Information

- Calories: 300
- Protein: 15g
- Carbohydrates: 30g
- Fat: 15g
- Fiber: 8g

Chia Seed Pudding with Blueberries and Almonds:

Cooking Time: Not Required | Serving: 1

Ingredients

- 1 serving = 1 serving
- 3 teaspoons of chia seeds
- 1 cup almond milk, unsweetened
- 1/2 cup blueberries, fresh
- 1 tbsp. slivered almonds
- a half teaspoon of vanilla extract

Preparation:

- ➢ Chia seeds, almond milk, and vanilla extract should be combined and refrigerated for many hours or overnight.
- ➢ Before serving, sprinkle with fresh blueberries and slivered almonds.

Nutritional Information

- Calories: 200
- Protein: 7g
- Carbohydrates: 20g
- Fat: 10g
- Fiber: 10g

Turkey and Sweet Potato Hash

Cooking Time: 10minute | **Serving: 1**

Ingredients

- 1/2 cup sweet potatoes, diced
- 2 ounces ground turkey
- 1/4 cup red bell pepper, diced
- 1/4 cup onion, diced
- 1 teaspoon olive oil

Preparation:

> In a skillet, sauté sweet potatoes, ground turkey, bell pepper, and onion in olive oil until cooked through.

Nutritional Information

- Calories: 250
- Protein: 15g
- Carbohydrates: 20g
- Fat: 12g
- Fiber: 5g

FLAVORFUL LUNCH

Salad with grilled chicken

Cooking Time: 15minutes | **Serving: 1**

Ingredients:

- ❖ 4 oz. skinless, boneless chicken breast
- ❖ 2 cups salad greens, mixed
- ❖ 1/2 cup halved cherry tomatoes
- ❖ 1/4 cup sliced cucumber
- ❖ 1 tablespoon extra virgin olive oil
- ❖ 1 tbsp. balsamic vinegar

Preparation:

- ✦ Season the chicken with salt and pepper and grill until cooked through.
- ✦ Salad greens, tomatoes, and cucumber should be combined.
- ✦ Place cooked chicken slices on top.
- ✦ Drizzle with balsamic vinegar and olive oil.

Nutritional Information

- Calories: 300
- Protein: 25g
- Carbohydrates: 10g
- Fat: 15g
- Fiber: 4g

Bowl of Quinoa and Black Beans

Cooking Time: 20minutes | **Serving: 1**

Ingredients

- ❖ 1/2 cup quinoa, cooked
- ❖ 1/2 cup black beans, drained and rinsed
- ❖ 1/4 cup corn kernels
- ❖ 1/4 cup bell peppers, diced
- ❖ 1 tablespoon extra virgin olive oil
- ❖ 1/2 teaspoon cumin

Preparation:

- Heat 1 tablespoon extra virgin olive oil over medium heat.
- Cook bell peppers and corn kernels for 2-3 minutes.
- Stir in cooked quinoa, sautéed veggies, and black beans.
- Combine quinoa, vegetables, and black beans in a mixing bowl.
- Sprinkle with 1/2 teaspoon cumin for uniform flavor dispersion.
- Fill a bowl halfway with quinoa and black bean mixture.
- Top with fresh cilantro, avocado slices, or lime juice if desired

Nutritional Information

- Calories: 250
- Protein: 12g
- Carbohydrates: 30g
- Fat: 8g
- Fiber:8g

Skewers with salmon and vegetables

Cooking Time: 15minutes | **Serving: 1**

Ingredients

- ❖ 4 oz. salmon fillet, cut into chunks
- ❖ 1/2 sliced zucchini
- ❖ 1/2 sliced red onion
- ❖ 1/2 chopped bell pepper
- ❖ 1 teaspoon of lemon juice
- ❖ 1 tablespoon of olive oil

Preparation:

- Combine salmon, lemon juice, and olive oil.
- Toss salmon evenly in the marinade.
- Allow 15 minutes for marinating.
- Cut zucchini, red onion, and bell pepper.
- Preheat grill or pan.
- Thread marinated salmon, vegetables, and skewers onto skewers.
- Place skewers on grill.

- ✚ Grill salmon for 3-4 minutes per side.
- ✚ Remove skewers and arrange on plate.
- ✚ Drizzle with additional lemon juice or oil for flavor.

Nutritional Information

- Calories: 300
- Protein: 20g
- Carbohydrates: 15g
- Fat: 18g
- Fiber: 4g

Soup with lentils and vegetables

Cooking Time: 30minutes | **Serving: 1**

Ingredients:

- ❖ 1/2 cup dried lentils,
- ❖ Rinsed 1 carrot,
- ❖ Diced 1 celery stalk,
- ❖ Diced 1/2 onion,
- ❖ Diced 2 cups low-sodium vegetable broth
- ❖ 1 tablespoon of olive oil

Preparation

- ✚ 1 tablespoon olive oil, heated in a pot over medium heat.
- ✚ To the pot, add the diced onion, carrot, and celery. Cook for 3-5 minutes, or until the vegetables soften.

Add the washed lentils and vegetable broth to the sautéed veggies in the pot.

- Bring the mixture to a boil, then reduce to a low heat, cover, and leave to simmer for 20-25 minutes, or until the lentils are cooked.

- After the lentils have finished cooking, taste the soup and adjust the seasoning as needed.
- If desired, top the lentil and vegetable soup with fresh herbs such as parsley or a squeeze of lemon juice

Nutritional Information

- Calories: 200
- Protein: 10g
- Carbohydrates: 30g
- Fat: 4g
- Fiber: 15g

Wrap with Turkey and Avocado

Cooking Time: 5minutes | Serving: 1

Ingredients:

- ❖ 3 oz. slices lean turkey
- ❖ 1 whole-wheat wrap
- ❖ 1/4 sliced avocado
- ❖ 1/2 cup shredded lettuce

❖ 1 teaspoon Greek yogurt

Preparation:

🔸 Wrap the turkey, avocado, and lettuce together.
🔸 Wrap in a wrap with Greek yogurt.

Nutritional Information

- calories:300
- protein:20g
- carbohydrate:25g
- Fat: 12g
- Fiber:8g

Tofu Stir-Fried with Vegetables

Cooking Time: 15minutes | Serving: 1

Ingredients:

❖ 4 oz. diced firm tofu
❖ 1 cup florets broccoli
❖ half a cup snap peas
❖ 1/2 sliced carrot
❖ 1 teaspoon of soy sauce
❖ 1 tbsp sesame oil

Preparation:

- In a wok or big skillet, heat 1 tablespoon sesame oil over medium-high heat.
- Stir-fry the chopped firm tofu in the heated oil for 2-3 minutes, or until it begins to become golden brown.
- To the tofu in the pan, add the broccoli florets, snap peas, and sliced carrot.
- Stir-fry for 4-5 minutes more, or until the vegetables are tender-crisp and the tofu is golden.
- 1 teaspoon soy sauce over the tofu and vegetables. To coat evenly, toss everything together.
- Remove the skillet from the heat once the tofu is thoroughly cooked and the vegetables are soft.
- Serve the Tofu Stir-Fry with Vegetables immediately, or over rice or noodles.

Nutritional Information

- calories:250
- protein:15g
- carbohydrates:20g
- Fat: 12g
- Fiber:8g

Stir-Fry with Chicken and Vegetables

Cooking Time: 15minutes | Serving: 1

Ingredients:

- 4 oz. cut chicken breast

- ❖ 1 cup mixed vegetables (carrots, bell peppers, broccoli)
- ❖ 1 tablespoon soy sauce (low sodium)
- ❖ 1 tablespoon extra virgin olive oil
- ❖ 1/2 teaspoon minced ginger

Preparation:

- Heat 1 tablespoon extra virgin olive oil in a large skillet or wok over medium-high heat. Stir-fry 4 oz. sliced chicken breast in the pan until it's cooked through and no longer pink in the center.
- Add 1 cup of mixed veggies to the skillet with the chicken, such as carrots, bell peppers, and broccoli. Stir-fry for another 3-5 minutes, or until the vegetables are tender-crisp
- Stir in 1/2 teaspoon minced ginger with the chicken and veggies in the pan.
- Finally, drizzle the mixture with 1 tablespoon of low-sodium soy sauce. Toss everything in the pan, making sure the soy sauce is well distributed.
- Stir-fry for another 1-2 minutes, or until everything is completely mixed and heated through.
- Serve your wonderful chicken and vegetable stir-fry immediately over rice or noodles, if desired. Have fun with your quick and easy stir-fry!

Nutritional Information

- Calories 300
- Protein:20g
  carbohydrate:1
  5g
- Fat: 15g
- Fiber: 6g

Salad with shrimp and avocado

Cooking Time: 10minutes | Serving: 1

Ingredients:

- ❖ 4 oz. peeled and deveined shrimp
- ❖ 1/2 avocado, sliced
- ❖ 2 cups salad greens, mixed
- ❖ 1/4 cup halved cherry tomatoes
- ❖ 1 tablespoon extra virgin olive oil

Preparation:

- ✛ Combine 4 oz. peeled and deveined shrimp, 1/2 sliced avocado, 2 cups mixed salad greens, and 1/4 cup halved cherry tomatoes in a medium-sized mixing dish. 1 tablespoon extra virgin olive oil should be drizzled over the items.

- Toss the shrimp, avocado, salad leaves, and tomatoes in the bowl with the olive oil, making sure the contents are uniformly coated.
- Serve the shrimp and avocado salad right away. For added flavor, add a bit of salt and pepper to taste, as well as a squeeze of fresh lemon or lime juice.

Nutritional Information

- Calories 250
- protein:20g
- carbohydrate:10g
- Fat: 15g
- Fiber:6g

Lemon and Herb Baked Cod

Cooking Time:15minutes| Serving:1

Ingredients

- ❖ 4 ounces of cod fillet
- ❖ 1 tablespoon extra virgin olive oil
- ❖ 1 tablespoon freshly squeezed lemon juice
- ❖ 1 teaspoon herb mixture (rosemary, thyme, parsley)

Preparation

- Preheat the oven to 400 degrees Fahrenheit (200 degrees Celsius).
- Place a 4-ounce fish fillet on a baking sheet that has been lightly oiled or coated with parchment paper.
- 1 tablespoon extra virgin olive oil, 1 tablespoon freshly squeezed lemon juice, and 1 teaspoon herb mixture (rosemary, thyme, parsley) in a small bowl.
- Brush the cod fillet with the olive oil, lemon, and herb mixture, making sure it's uniformly coated on both sides.
- Bake the cod for 12-15 minutes, or until opaque and flaky with a fork, in a preheated oven.
- Serve your cooked cod with lemon and herb with your favorite side dishes. Enjoy your wonderful and nutritious dish!

.Nutritional Information

- Calories 200
- protein:20g
- carbohydrate:2g
- Fat: 12g
- Fiber:1g

Stew with Eggplant and Chickpeas

Cooking Time: 20minutes | **Serving: 1**

Ingredients:

* 1 cup sliced eggplant
* 1/2 cup cleaned and drained canned chickpeas
* 1/2 cup tomato dice
* 1/4 cup chopped onion
* 1 minced garlic clove
* 1 tablespoon of olive oil

Preparation

* Heat 1 tablespoon olive oil in a medium-sized pot over medium heat. To the pot, add 1/4 cup chopped onion and 1 minced garlic clove. Sauté the onions and garlic until transparent and aromatic.
* Cook for a few minutes, until the eggplant begins to soften, with 1 cup of sliced eggplant.
* Add 1/2 cup cleaned and drained canned chickpeas and 1/2 cup diced tomatoes and mix well.
* Cover the pot and cook over low to medium heat for 15-20 minutes, or until the eggplant is soft and the flavors have mingled.
* Season to taste with salt and pepper.
* Serve your eggplant and chickpea stew hot, garnished if desired with fresh herbs such as parsley or cilantro.

Nutritional Information

* calories 250
* protein:10g
* carbohydrates:30g
* Fat: 10g

66

Skillet with Turkey and Vegetables

Cooking Time: 15minutes | Serving:1

Ingredients:

- ❖ 4 ounces ground turkey
- ❖ 1/2 cup sliced zucchini
- ❖ 1/2 cup diced bell pepper
- ❖ 1/4 cup minced onion
- ❖ 1 tablespoon of olive oil

Preparation:

- ┿ Heat 1 tablespoon olive oil in a pan over medium-high heat.
- ┿ Cook until browned, breaking it apart with a spoon as it cooks, in a skillet with 4 ounces of turkey.
- ┿ After the turkey has been browned, add 1/2 cup sliced zucchini, 1/2 cup diced bell pepper, and 1/4 cup chopped onion to the skillet.
- ┿ Cook for a further 5-7 minutes, or until the veggies are soft and the turkey is fully cooked, stirring occasionally.

+ Season the skillet with salt and pepper to taste, or any other ingredients you choose.
+ Serve your turkey and veggie skillet hot, garnished if desired with fresh herbs such as parsley or cilantro.

Nutritional Information

- calories 300
- protein: 20g
- carbohydrate:15g
- Fat: 15g
- Fiber:4g

Chicken Breast with Spinach and Feta Stuffing
Cooking Time: 25minutes | Serving: 1

Ingredients

- 1 skinless, boneless chicken breast
- 1 cup fresh spinach
- 1/4 cup crumbled feta cheese
- 1 garlic clove chopped
- 1 tablespoon olive oil

Preparation

+ Preheat the oven to 375 degrees Fahrenheit (190 degrees Celsius).

- In a small mixing dish, combine 1 cup fresh spinach, 1/4 cup crumbled feta cheese, and 1 minced garlic clove.
- Make a pocket in the side of the skinless, boneless chicken breast using a sharp knife. Make sure you don't cut all the way through.
- Stuff the spinach and feta mixture into the chicken breast pocket you made.
- Heat 1 tablespoon olive oil in an oven-safe skillet over medium-high heat.
- Sear the stuffed chicken breast in the skillet for 2-3 minutes on each side, or until golden brown.
- Bake for 20-25 minutes, or until the chicken is cooked through and reaches an internal temperature of 165°F (74°C), in a preheated oven.
- Serve your tasty chicken breast with spinach and feta stuffing hot, decorated with fresh herbs or a squeeze of lemon if wanted

Nutritional Information

calories 250
protein:30g
carbohydrate:5g
Fat: ~12g
Fiber:2g

Caprese Salad with Grilled Chicken

Cooking Time: 15minutes | Serving: 1

Ingredients:

- ❖ 4 ounces grilled chicken breast
- ❖ 1 cup halved cherry tomatoes
- ❖ 1/2 cup diced fresh mozzarella
- ❖ 1 tablespoon balsamic glaze
- ❖ 1/4 cup fresh basil leaves

Preparation:

- Grill the chicken breast until cooked through, then cut it into bite-sized pieces.
- Cut the cherry tomatoes in half.
- Make tiny cubes of fresh mozzarella.
- Collect fresh basil leaves.
- Combine the grilled chicken slices, split cherry tomatoes, diced fresh mozzarella, and fresh basil leaves in a large mixing dish.
- Drizzle 1 tablespoon balsamic glaze over the bowl's contents.
- To provide a uniform coating of the balsamic glaze and to blend the flavors, gently toss the contents in the bowl.
- Garnish with additional fresh basil leaves or a sprinkling of black pepper if preferred..

Nutritional Information

- calories 300
- Protein: 25g
- Carbohydrates: 10g
- Fat: ~15g
- fiber:5g

Vegetable and Quinoa Stuffed Pepper

Cooking Time: 30minutes | Serving: 1

Ingredients:

- 2 halved bell peppers
- 1/2 cup cooked quinoa
- 1/2 cup drained and rinsed black beans
- 1/4 cup kernel corn
- 1/4 cup diced tomatoes
- 1/4 cup diced red onion
- 1 teaspoon olive oil

Preparation

- Preheat the oven to 375 degrees Fahrenheit (190 degrees Celsius).
- Combine cooked quinoa, black beans, kernel corn, diced tomatoes, diced red onion, and olive oil in a mixing dish.

71

+ Stuff the quinoa and vegetable mixture into the half
  bell peppers.
+ Place the stuffed peppers on a baking sheet and
  bake for 20-25 minutes, or until tender.
+ Have fun with your Vegetable and Quinoa Stuffed
  Peppers!

Nutritional Information

- Calories: 250
- Protein: 10g
- Carbohydrates: 40g
- Fat: 5g
- Fiber: 8g

Asian-Inspired Salmon Bowl:

Cooking Time: 20minutes | Serving: 1

Ingredients:

- ❖ 4 oz. salmon fillet
- ❖ 1/2 cup broccoli florets
- ❖ 1/2 cup snow peas
- ❖ 1/2 cup cooked brown rice
- ❖ 1 tbsp low-sodium soy sauce
- ❖ Half a teaspoon sesame oil

Preparation

- Cook the 4 oz. salmon fillet in a pan until it's done to your preference.
- Stir-fry broccoli florets and snow peas in the same pan until tender-crisp.
- Serve the cooked salmon over cooked brown rice with the stir-fried broccoli and snow peas.
- Drizzle 1 tbsp low-sodium soy sauce and 1/2 teaspoon sesame oil over the bowl.
- Enjoy your simple and tasty Asian-Inspired Salmon Bowl!

Nutritional Information

- Calories: 300
- Protein: 25g
- Carbohydrates: 30g
- Fat: 12g
- Fiber: 5g

CHAPTER FIVE

FLAVORFUL DINNER

Grilled Lemon Herb Chicken

Cooking Time: 20minutes | Serving: 1

Ingredients:

- 4 skinless, boneless chicken breasts
- 2 tbsp of olive oil
- 1 tablespoon freshly squeezed lemon juice
- 1 tsp. dried oregano
- 1 tsp. garlic powder
- Season with salt and pepper to taste

Preparation:

- Combine the olive oil, lemon juice, oregano, garlic powder, salt, and pepper in a mixing bowl.
- Marinate the chicken breasts for 30 minutes in the mixture.
- Grill for 15-20 minutes, rotating once or twice, until completely done.

Nutritional Information:

- Calories: 250
- Protein: 30g
- Carbohydrates: 1g
- Fat: 12g

Baked Salmon with Dill

Cooking Time: 20minutes | Serving: 1

Ingredients:

- 4 fillets of salmon
- 2 tbsp of olive oil
- 1 tablespoon chopped fresh dill
- 1 tsp. lemon zest
- Season with salt and pepper to taste.

Preparation:

- Preheat the oven to 375 degrees Fahrenheit (190 degrees Celsius).
- On a baking sheet, place the salmon fillets.
- Spread olive oil, dill, lemon zest, salt, and pepper on top of the fish.
- Bake for 15-20 minutes, or until the fish is readily flakes.

Nutritional Information:

- Calories: 300
- Protein: 25g
- Carbohydrates: 0g
- Fat: 20g

Quinoa and Vegetable Stir-Fry

Cooking Time: 15minutes | Serving: 1

Ingredients:

- 1 cup cooked quinoa
- 1 cup florets broccoli
- 1 finely sliced bell pepper
- 1 julienned carrot
- 2 tbsp. low-sodium soy sauce
- 1 tablespoon extra virgin olive oil

Preparation:

- ➢ Rinse 1 cup of quinoa and cook according to package directions.
- ➢ Cut broccoli into florets, slice bell pepper and carrot, and heat 1 tablespoon of extra virgin olive oil in a large skillet. Cook the vegetables until softened but crisp.
- ➢ Add cooked quinoa and vegetables, then pour 2 tablespoons of low-sodium soy sauce over them. Stir-fry for 2-3 minutes until well coated.
- ➢ Remove from heat and serve warm.

Nutritional Information:

- Calories: 300
- Protein: 10g
- Carbohydrates: 45g
- Fat: 8g

Turkey and Vegetable Skewers

Cooking Time: 20minutes | Serving: 2 skewers

Ingredients:

- 1 pound turkey breast, cubed
- 1 sliced zucchini
- 1 red onion, peeled and diced
- 1 tablespoon extra virgin olive oil
- 1 teaspoon thyme dried

Preparation:

➢ Mix turkey breast, zucchini, red onion, olive oil, thyme, salt, and pepper.
➢ Thread onto skewers, grill or bake at 400°F.
➢ Cook for 10-15 minutes or until turkey is cooked through.
➢ Bake for 20-25 minutes. Serve hot, garnished with herbs or lemon if desired..

Nutritional Information:

- Calories: 280
- Protein: 30g
- Carbohydrates: 5g
- Fat: 14g

Eggplant and Chickpea Curry

Cooking time: 25minutes | **Serving: 1**

Ingredients:

- 1 diced eggplant
- 1 can chickpeas, drained
- 1 onion, minced
- 2 diced tomatoes
- 2 teaspoons curry powder
- 1 cup veggie broth

Preparation:

- Combine chopped eggplant, drained chickpeas, minced onion, diced tomatoes, curry powder, and veggie broth in a large pan or saucepan.
- Over medium heat, bring the mixture to a simmer.
- Allow it to cook for 15-20 minutes, or until the eggplant is soft and the flavors have blended properly.

➢ After cooking, serve the Eggplant and Chickpea Curry over rice or with your favorite bread.

Nutritional Information:

- Calories: 250
- Protein: 10g
- Carbohydrates: 45g
- Fat: 5g

Shrimp and Asparagus Stir-Fry

Cooking Time: 15minutes | Serving: 1

Ingredients:

- 1 pound peeled and deveined shrimp
- 1 asparagus bunch, trimmed and sliced into 2-inch pieces
- 2 tbsp. low-sodium soy sauce
- 1 tbsp sesame seed oil
- 1 teaspoon minced ginger

Preparation:

➢ Heat sesame seed oil in a wok or big skillet over medium-high heat.

- ➢ Stir-fry the peeled and deveined shrimp in the heated pan for about 2 minutes, or until they start to become pink and opaque.
- ➢ Add sliced asparagus to the pan with the shrimp.
- ➢ Stir-fry for 3-4 minutes more, or until the shrimp are thoroughly cooked and the asparagus is tender-crisp.
- ➢ In the last minute of cooking, add the minced ginger to the pan and swirl to combine.
- ➢ Over the shrimp and asparagus, drizzle with low-sodium soy sauce. Toss everything together for 1-2 minutes more, making sure the tastes are fully integrated.
- ➢ Remove the skillet from the heat once the shrimp are thoroughly cooked and the asparagus is soft.
- ➢ Serve the Shrimp and Asparagus Stir-Fry immediately over rice or noodles.

Nutritional Information:

- • Calories: 220
- • Protein: 25g
- • Carbohydrates: 7g
- • Fat: 10g

Spinach and Feta Stuffed Chicken

Cooking Time: 30minutes | Serving: 1

Ingredients:

- 4 breasts of chicken
- 2 cups spinach, fresh
- 1/2 cup crumbled feta cheese
- 1 tsp. dried basil
- Season with salt and pepper to taste.

Preparation:

- Preheat the oven to 375 degrees Fahrenheit (190 degrees Celsius).
- Combine fresh spinach, crumbled feta cheese, dried basil, salt, and pepper in a mixing bowl.
- Make a pocket in each chicken breast with a sharp knife by cutting horizontally along one side, being careful not to cut through the other.
- Stuff the spinach and feta mixture inside each chicken breast.
- Season the outside of each packed chicken breast to taste with salt and pepper.
- In a baking dish, place the filled chicken breasts.
- Bake for 25-30 minutes, or until the chicken is cooked through and no longer pink in the center, in a preheated oven.
- When the stuffed chicken is done, remove it from the oven and let it aside for a few minutes before serving.

➤ Serve the Spinach and Feta Stuffed Chicken hot, garnished with fresh herbs or a squeeze of lemon if desired.

Nutritional Information:

- Calories: 280
- Protein: 30g
- Carbohydrates: 2g
- Fat: 16g

Lentil and Vegetable Soup

Cooking Time:40minutes | **Serving: 2**

Ingredients:

- 1 cup washed dry green lentils
- 1 onion, chopped
- 2 carrots, sliced
- 2 cut celery stalks
- 4 cups veggie broth
- 1 tablespoon cumin
- Season with salt and pepper to taste.

Preparation:

➤ In a large pot, combine washed dry green lentils, chopped onion, sliced carrots, celery stalks, veggie broth, cumin, and season with salt and pepper to taste.

- ➢ Cook until lentils and veggies are soft.

Nutritional Information:

- Calories: 220
- Protein: 15g
- Carbohydrates: 40g
- Fat: 2g

Roasted Vegetable Medley

Cooking Time: 35minutes | Serving: 1

Ingredients:

- 2 cups halved Brussels sprouts
- 2 cups florets cauliflower
- 1 diced sweet potato
- 2 tbsp of olive oil
- 1 teaspoon thyme
- Season with salt and pepper to taste.

Preparation:

- ➢ Preheat the oven to the desired roasting temperature (often 400°F or 200°C).
- ➢ Combine 2 cups halved Brussels sprouts, 2 cups cauliflower florets, and 1 diced sweet potato in a mixing basin.
- ➢ Toss the vegetables with 2 tablespoons olive oil, 1 teaspoon thyme, and season to taste with salt and

pepper. Spread the seasoned vegetables on a baking sheet and roast until golden and soft in a preheated oven.

Nutritional Information:

- Calories: 180
- Protein: 5g
- Carbohydrates: 30g
- Fat: 7g

Greek Salad with Grilled Chicken

Cooking Time: 20minutes | Serving: 1

Ingredients:

- 2 cups salad greens, mixed
- 1 cucumber, sliced
- 1 cup cherry tomatoes, halved
- 1/2 cup crumbled feta cheese
- 2 tbsp olive oil
- 1 grilled chicken breast, sliced
- 1 tbsp. red wine vinegar

Preparation:

➤ Combine 2 cups mixed salad greens, sliced cucumber, halved cherry tomatoes, and 1/2 cup crumbled feta cheese in a large mixing basin.

> Drizzle 2 tablespoons olive oil and 1 tablespoon red wine vinegar over the salad. To coat the salad uniformly, toss the ingredients together.
> Serve the salad with grilled chicken breast slices on top. Serve right away for a delectable Greek Salad with Grilled Chicken.

Nutritional Information:

- Calories: 300
- Protein: 25g
- Carbohydrates: 10g
- Fat: 18g

Baked Cod with Lemon and Herbs

Cooking Time: 25minutes | Serving: 1

Ingredients:

- 4 fillets of cod
- 2 tbsp. softened butter
- 1 sliced lemon
- 1 teaspoon thyme dried
- Season with salt and pepper to taste.

Preparation:

> Preheat the oven to the required baking temperature, which is usually approximately 375°F (190°C).

85

➢ Arrange the cod fillets on a baking sheet. Spread 2 tablespoons melted butter over the fillets and top with 1 teaspoon dry thyme. Season to taste with salt and pepper. Place lemon wedges on top of each fillet.

➢ Bake for 15-20 minutes, or until the fish is cooked through and flakes readily with a fork, in a preheated oven. Serve the Baked Cod with Lemon and Herbs immediately, if preferred garnished with additional lemon slices.

Nutritional Information

- Calories: 220
- Protein: 30g
- Carbohydrates: 0g
- Fat: 10g

Zucchini Noodles with Pesto

Cooking Time: 15minutes | Serving:1

Ingredients:

- 4 spiralized medium zucchini
- 1/2 cup halved cherry tomatoes
- 2 teaspoons pesto sauce
- 1 tbsp Parmesan cheese, grated

Preparation:

➢ Cook until the zucchini noodles are soft.

➢ Toss with pesto and cherry tomatoes.

➢ Before serving, sprinkle with Parmesan cheese.

Nutritional Information:

- Calories: 180
- Protein: 5g
- Carbohydrates: 15g
- Fat: 12g

Stuffed Bell Peppers with Turkey and Quinoa

Cooking Time: 30minutes | Serving: 2

Ingredients:

- 4 halved bell peppers
- 1 pound ground turkey
- 1 cup quinoa, cooked
- 1 can drained black beans
- 1 quart salsa
- 1 tablespoon cumin
- Season with salt and pepper to taste.

Preparation:

➢ Preheat the oven to 375 degrees Fahrenheit (190 degrees Celsius).
➢ Combine ground turkey, cooked quinoa, drained black beans, salsa, and 1 tablespoon cumin in a large mixing dish. Season the mixture to taste with salt and pepper. Combine thoroughly.
➢ Fill each divided bell pepper half with the turkey-quinoa mixture. Place the stuffed peppers in a baking dish, cover with foil, and bake for about 25-30 minutes, or until the peppers are soft. Serve the Stuffed Bell Peppers with Turkey and Quinoa hot, garnished with more salsa and fresh herbs if desired.

Nutritional Information:

- Calories: 280
- Protein: 25g
- Carbohydrates: 30g
- Fat: 8g

Chicken and Vegetable Curry

Cooking Time: 25minutes | Serving: 1

Ingredients:

- 1 pound boneless and skinless chicken thighs
- 1 chopped onion
- 2 sliced bell peppers

- 1 can coconut milk
- Two tbsp curry powder
- Season with salt and pepper to taste.

Preparation:

- Cook 1 pound of boneless, skinless chicken thighs in a large skillet or pot over medium heat until browned. Take the chicken out of the pan and set it aside.
- Sauté the chopped onion in the same skillet until transparent. Continue to sauté the sliced bell peppers until they are slightly softened.
- Return the cooked chicken to the skillet, add the coconut milk, and season with 2 teaspoons curry powder. Season to taste with salt and pepper. Simmer the mixture over medium-low heat for 15-20 minutes, or until the chicken is cooked through and the flavors have melded.
- Serve the Chicken and Vegetable Curry over rice or with your favorite side dish..

Nutritional Information:

- Calories: 320
- Protein: 20g
- Carbohydrates: 10g
- Fat: 22g

Broccoli and Mushroom Frittata

Cooking Time: 25minutes | **Serving:** 1/6th of the frittata

Ingredients:

- 6 eggs
- 1 cup steamed broccoli florets
- 1 cup sliced mushrooms
- 1/2 cup shredded Swiss cheese
- Season with salt and pepper to taste.

Preparation:

- Preheat the broiler in your oven.
- 6 eggs should be whisked together in a mixing bowl. Steamed broccoli florets, sliced mushrooms, and 1/2 cup shredded Swiss cheese are added last. Season the mixture to taste with salt and pepper.
- Pour the egg and vegetable mixture into an oven-safe skillet that has been warmed. Cook for a few minutes over medium heat until the sides are firm, then place the skillet under the broiler. Broil for 2-3 minutes more, or until the top is golden brown and the frittata is thoroughly cooked. Serve your scrumptious Broccoli and Mushroom Frittata in slices.

Nutritional Information:

- Calories: 250
- Protein: 15g
- Carbohydrates: 5g
- Fat: 18g

SNACKS IDEAS

Greek Yogurt Parfait

Ingredients:

- ✓ 1 cup plain Greek yogurt
- ✓ 1/2 cup fresh berries (strawberries, blueberries, etc.)
- ✓ 1 tablespoon chopped nuts (almonds, walnuts, etc.)
- ✓ 1 teaspoon (optional) honey

Preparation:

- Layer Greek yogurt, berries, and nuts in a bowl or glass.
- If desired, drizzle with honey.

Nutritional Information:

Calories: 200 | Protein: 15g | Carbohydrates: 20g |

Fat: 8g

Serving Size: 1 parfait

Vegetable Sticks with Hummus

Ingredients:

- ✓ 1 cup carrots, baby
- ✓ 1 cup sliced cucumber
- ✓ hummus (two tablespoons)

Preparation:

- On a platter, arrange carrot and cucumber sticks.
- Serve alongside hummus for dipping.

Nutritional Information:

Calories: 150 | Protein: 4g | Carbohydrates: 15g | Fat: 8g

Serving Size: 1 cup of veggies with hummus

Almond and Cheese Platter

Ingredients:

- ✓ 1 cup almonds
- ✓ 1 ounce cheese (such as cheddar or mozzarella)
- ✓ 1 pound cherry tomatoes

Preparation:

- On a dish, arrange the almonds, cheese, and cherry tomatoes.

Nutritional Information:

Calories: 250 | Protein: 12g | Carbohydrates: 6g | Fat: 20g

Serving Size: 1 platter

Cottage Cheese and Pineapple Bowl

Ingredients:

- ✓ 1/2 cup cottage cheese (low-fat)
- ✓ 1/2 cup pineapple chunks, fresh
- ✓ 1 tbsp. sunflower seeds

Preparation:

- ⬥ In a mixing dish, combine cottage cheese and pineapple.
- ⬥ Sunflower seeds can be sprinkled on top.

Nutritional Information:

Calories: 180 | Protein: 15g | Carbohydrates: 20g | Fat: 5g

Serving Size: 1 bowl

Avocado and Tomato Salsa

Ingredients:

- ✓ 1 ripe avocado, diced
- ✓ 1/2 cup cherry tomatoes, diced
- ✓ 1 tablespoon red onion, coarsely minced
- ✓ 1 tablespoon cilantro, chopped

Preparation:

- ⬥ Combine avocado, tomatoes, red onion, cilantro, and lime juice in a mixing bowl.
- ⬥ Gently combine and serve with whole-grain crackers.

Nutritional Information:

Calories: 180 | Protein: 3g | Carbohydrates: 12g | Fat: 14g

Serving Size: 1 cup of salsa with crackers

Hard-Boiled Eggs with Mustard

Ingredients:

- ✓ 2 eggs, hard-boiled
- ✓ 1 tbsp. Dijon mustard
- ✓ Season with salt and pepper to taste.

Preparation:

- Hard-boiled eggs, cut in half.
- Season with salt and pepper on each side with mustard.

Nutritional Information:

Calories: 160 | Protein: 14g | Carbohydrates:2g | Fat: 11g

Serving Size: 2 egg halves

Tuna Salad Lettuce Wraps

Ingredients:

- ✓ 1 drained can tuna
- ✓ 2 tbsp mayonnaise (mild preferred)
- ✓ 1 finely sliced celery stalk
- ✓ Salt and pepper to taste
- ✓ Lettuce leaves for wrapping

Preparation:

- Combine tuna, mayonnaise, celery, salt, and pepper in a mixing bowl.
- Wrap the tuna mixture with lettuce leaves.

Nutritional Information:

Calories: 180 | Protein: 20g | Carbohydrates: 2g | Fat: 10g

Serving Size: 1 serving of wraps

Cherry Almond Energy Bites

Ingredients:

- ✓ 1 cup drained dried cherries
- ✓ 1 pound almonds
- ✓ 1 teaspoon chia seeds
- ✓ A tsp vanilla extract

Preparation:

- Blend cherries, almonds, chia seeds, and vanilla extract in a food processor until finely chopped.
- Refrigerate after rolling into bite-sized balls.

Nutritional Information:

Calories: 150 | Protein: 4g | Carbohydrates: 15g | Fat: 9g

Serving Size: 2 energy bites

Edamame Snack Bowl

Ingredients:

- ✓ 1 cup steamed edamame
- ✓ 1 tbsp sesame oil
- ✓ 1 teaspoon of sea salt

Preparation:

- ♣ Steamed edamame should be tossed with sesame oil and sea salt.

Nutritional Information:

Calories: 120 | Protein: 11g | Carbohydrates: 8g | Fat: 6g

Serving Size: 1 cup

Berry and Nut Smoothie

Ingredients:

- ✓ 1/2 cup mixed berries (strawberries, blueberries, etc.)
- ✓ a quarter cup almonds
- ✓ 1 cup almond milk, unsweetened
- ✓ 1 teaspoon flaxseed

Preparation:

- ♣ Blend till smooth the mixed berries, almonds, almond milk, and flaxseeds.

Nutritional Information:

Calories: 200 | Protein: 7g | Carbohydrates: 15g | Fat: 12g

Serving Size: 1 smoothie

FLAVORFUL DESSERT

Baked Apple with Cinnamon

Ingredients:

- ✓ 2 cored medium-sized apples
- ✓ 1 teaspoon ground cinnamon
- ✓ 1 tbsp. chopped walnuts
- ✓ 1 tablespoon honey (optional).

Preparation:

- ✦ Preheat the oven to 375 degrees Fahrenheit (190 degrees Celsius).
- ✦ Arrange the cored apples on a baking pan.
- ✦ Fill the core with chopped walnuts and sprinkle with cinnamon.
- ✦ Cook for 20–25 minutes.
- ✦ If desired, drizzle with honey.

Nutritional Information:

Calories: 150 | Protein: 2g | Carbohydrates: 30g | Fat: 4g

Serving Size: 1 apple

Berries and Cream Parfait

Ingredients:

✓ 1 cup mixed berries (strawberries, blueberries, etc.)
✓ 1/2 cup unsweetened Greek yogurt
✓ 1 tbsp. chopped almonds
✓ a tsp vanilla extract

Preparation:

+ Layer mixed berries, Greek yogurt, and sliced almonds in a glass.
+ Layers should be repeated.
+ Drizzle with vanilla extract to finish.

Nutritional Information:

Calories: 180 | Protein: 12g | Carbohydrates: 20g | Fat: 7g

Serving Size: 1 parfait

Dark Chocolate-Dipped Strawberries

Ingredients:

✓ 8 large cleaned and dried strawberries
✓ 2 ounces dark chocolate (70% cocoa or higher)

Preparation:

+ In a heatproof basin, melt the dark chocolate.
+ Each strawberry should be dipped into the melted chocolate.
+ Refrigerate on a parchment-lined tray until the chocolate sets.

Nutritional Information:

Calories: 120 Protein: 2g Carbohydrates: 15g Fat: 7g

Serving Size: 2 strawberries

Chia Seed Pudding

Ingredients:

- ✓ 2 tbsp of chia seeds
- ✓ 1 cup almond milk, unsweetened
- ✓ a half teaspoon of vanilla extract
- ✓ 1/2 cup berries, mixed

Preparation:

- In a mixing dish, combine the chia seeds, almond milk, and vanilla essence.
- Refrigerate for at least two hours, preferably overnight.
- Before serving, sprinkle with mixed berries.

Nutritional Information:

Calories: 150 Protein: 5g Carbohydrates: 15g Fat: 8g

Serving Size: 1 cup

Frozen Yogurt Bites

Ingredients:

✓ 1 cup unsweetened Greek yogurt

✓ 1 tablespoon honey 1/2 cup chopped mixed berries

Preparation:

- In a mixing bowl, combine Greek yogurt, sliced berries, and honey.
- Fill small silicone molds halfway with the mixture.
- Freeze for 2-3 hours, or until firm.

Nutritional Information:

Calories: 120 | Protein: 8g | Carbohydrates: 15g | Fat: 4g

Serving Size: 2-3 bites

Cinnamon Baked Pears

Ingredients:

- ✓ 2 peeled and cored ripe pears
- ✓ 1 teaspoon ground cinnamon
- ✓ 1 tbsp. chopped pecans
- ✓ 1 teaspoon (optional) honey

Preparation:

- Preheat the oven to 375 degrees Fahrenheit (190 degrees Celsius).
- Arrange the pear halves on a baking sheet.
- Sprinkle with cinnamon and nuts, if desired.
- Cook for 20–25 minutes.

↓ If desired, drizzle with honey.

Nutritional Information:

Calories: 160 | Protein: 2g | Carbohydrates: 30g | Fat: 6g

Serving Size: 1 pear

Avocado Chocolate Mousse

Ingredients:

- ✓ 2 avocados, ripe
- ✓ 1/4 cup chocolate powder, unsweetened
- ✓ a quarter cup almond milk
- ✓ 2 teaspoons honey
- ✓ a tsp vanilla extract

Preparation:

- ↓ Smoothly combine avocados, cocoa powder, almond milk, honey, and vanilla extract.
- ↓ Refrigerate for at least one hour before serving.

Nutritional Information:

Calories: 200 | Protein: 3g | Carbohydrates: 20g | Fat: 15g

Serving Size: 1/2 cup

Pumpkin Spice Baked Apples

Ingredients:

- ✓ 2 cored medium-sized apples
- ✓ 2 teaspoons pureed pumpkin
- ✓ 1 teaspoon pumpkin pie spice
- ✓ 1 tbsp. chopped pecans

Preparation:

- Preheat the oven to 375 degrees Fahrenheit (190 degrees Celsius).
- Arrange the cored apples on a baking pan.
- Combine pumpkin puree and pumpkin spice in a mixing basin.
- Fill apple cores with pumpkin mixture and sprinkle with pecans.
- 20-25 minutes in the oven.

Nutritional Information:

Calories: 180 | Protein: 2g | Carbohydrates: 30g | Fat: 8g

Serving Size: 1 apple

Coconut Almond Balls

Ingredients:

- ✓ 1 cup edamame, steamed
- ✓ 1 teaspoon sesame oil
- ✓ 1/2 teaspoon sea salt .

Preparation:

- ✦ Combine shredded coconut, almond meal, melted coconut oil, almond butter, and vanilla essence in a mixing dish.
- ✦ Refrigerate for 1 hour after shaping into tiny balls.

Nutritional Information:

| Calories: 120 | Protein: 3g | Carbohydrates: 5g | Fat: 10g |

Serving Size: 2 balls

Raspberry Almond Tartlets

Ingredients:

- ✓ 1 casserole almond flour
- ✓ 2 teaspoons melted coconut oil
- ✓ 1 teaspoon honey
- ✓ 1 pound fresh raspberries

Preparation:

reheat the oven to 350°F/175°C.

Combine almond flour, melted coconut oil, and honey in a mixing bowl.

Fill tartlet molds with the mixture.

Bake for 15-20 minutes, then top with fresh raspberries.

Nutritional Information:

Calories: 150 | Protein: 5g | Carbohydrates: 10g | Fat: 10g

Serving Size: 2 tartlets

CONCLUSION

In conclusion, adopting a diabetic-friendly diet for people over 50 is a proactive and powerful step in managing and preventing diabetes complications. The recipes presented are not only customized to fulfill the nutritional demands of seniors, but they are also delicious and varied, ensuring that eating a balanced diet is a pleasurable experience.

The concentration on lean proteins, whole grains, and fiber-rich fruits and vegetables supports steady blood sugar levels, which helps to reduce spikes and crashes, which can be especially difficult for diabetics. These recipes also include nutrient-dense products, which promote overall health and well-being as well as diabetic management.

Furthermore, the recipes' adaptability allows for culinary discovery, making it easier for people to follow a diabetic-friendly diet without compromising flavor or variety. There are a variety of options to accommodate different tastes and preferences, ranging from grilled lemon herb chicken to chia seed pudding.

As you embark on this culinary adventure, keep in mind that tiny, long-term adjustments can have a big influence on your health. It is not just about managing diabetes; it is also about adopting a healthy lifestyle. Every meal is an opportunity to fuel your body and develop habits that will help you live a long and healthy life.

Consider this trip as an investment in your future in the spirit of fostering a better you. Celebrate the positive changes, savor the flavors, and be grateful for the attention you're giving your body. Your dedication to a diabetic-friendly diet is a significant act of self-love and resilience. You are taking ownership of your health and embracing the opportunity to live your best, most vibrant life by adopting and adjusting to these recipes. Remember that every healthful choice you make is a step toward a healthier, happier you.